Alzheimer’
Memory Book

Caregivers Design Guide

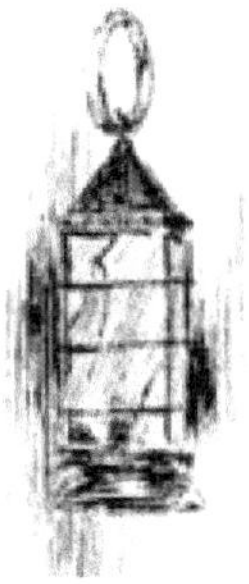

Introduction

Have you ever looked at pictures with someone and said: "Look at this! Do you remember that Halloween when..." If you have, then you were using your memory. Maybe you've looked at a picture of an Aunt who went parasailing when she was 76, and said: "Do you remember Aunt Alice? Look at this picture!" Again, you were using your memory.

As Alzheimer's disease progresses those who are afflicted will lose their memories. Health care professionals have divided the symptoms of Alzheimer's disease into two categories: "Cognitive" and "behavioral and psychiatric". It is the "cognitive" aspect of this disease that I'm addressing here as a caregiver. It was our observation that our "Memory Book" did indeed seem to help our dear family member.

Sometimes the onset of Alzheimer's is gradual, and sometimes it's rapid. With a healthy diet, prescriptions, and memory exercises this disease can likely be slowed. This would allow an individual to maintain a higher quality of life for a longer period of time.

Memory exercises do not have to be complex. In fact, by observing just one photograph it appears that our memory can bring back many related experiences. You know this is true because it's happened to you, right? Having the ability to bring these memories back to mind each day is a mental exercise healthy people don't even think twice about. I found that this "photographic recall" appeared to be a good mental exercise, and was helpful in bringing additional memories back to someone afflicted with Alzheimer's. This was clearly apparent in the nonverbal expression as the individual reviewed the photos.

This benefit seemed to work for us, and this systematic approach was developed which is the focus of this book.

Best regards in your care giving. Remember to take some time for yourself. You deserve it!

The Author

Table of Contents

This book is dedicated to...

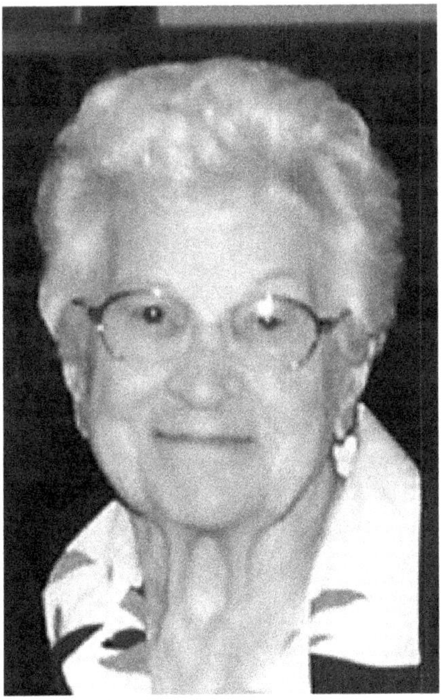

Carol May Jenkinson
1917 – 2008

Chapter 1

Discovery

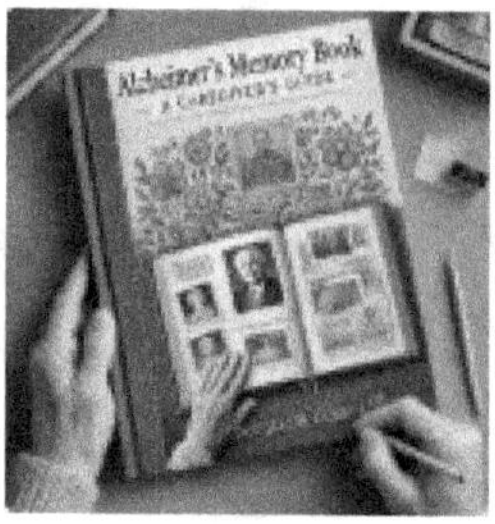

My wife and I were caregivers for her mother, Carol, who was first diagnosed with Alzheimer's at age 85. We learned that Carol had Alzheimer's quite by accident. You see, Carol and my wife shared the same doctor. One day while at a routine yearly checkup, my wife's doctor asked in casual conversation how her mother's Alzheimer's was progressing. Of course this was rather shocking, since Carol "forgot" to mention it. By this time about 2 years had passed since the doctor had diagnosed Carol with the disease. Carol didn't drive, and was living alone at that time. Although someone had to drive Carol to and from the doctor's appointments during this two year time period, the driver waited in the office lobby, they never actually went in to see the Doctor with Carol. Therefore, none of the family became aware of her condition. Compounding this is the fact that it wasn't necessarily the same person each time that would drive Carol to the doctor's appointment!

In hind sight, I imagine that the doctor wasn't actually obligated to share Carol's diagnosis. Perhaps, there are also legal reasons involved here, which are likely different from state to state. If the coincidence of sharing the same physician with my wife wasn't held in common, then it may have been only when Carol's Alzheimer's Disease had critically progressed, that the family would have learned of this most serious condition. So began our arrival into the world of Alzheimer's.

When do the Alzheimer's symptoms begin to show, to where other people would recognize that something isn't quite right? That would be in late Stage 2 in my opinion. At least in Carol's case I believe this was true. Of course my question has always been: what brought the Doctor's attention to diagnose Carol's AD in the first place? We never learned the answer to that. We are just grateful that it was brought to our attention when it was. You see Carol lived alone, although she had frequent company. But, the same people wouldn't see her every day. With four sons, a daughter, and adult grandchildren she had a good many people visit her throughout the week. Yet, no one would have noticed that something had changed, that something was wrong, unless they were with her daily. From talking with others who have loved one's with Alzheimer's, I think the answer to "when symptoms would show" also depends on the individual's personality. Some individuals can "hide" the Alzheimer's in its early stages to prevent it from "showing" to others. After all, forgetting things can be embarrassing.

Maybe, Carol was having trouble balancing her check book, and mentioned that to her doctor. This could well have initiated the diagnosis. She would not be inclined to bring the check book issue to someone until it was too late. And, looking back on it now, that's just what happened. Carol asked my wife to look at her check book for her. It was just a short while after that when the routine Doctor's visit occurred, and the Alzheimer's was brought up in casual conversation.

Although there are several methods that the medical experts have developed to categorize the key symptoms of Alzheimer's, my wife and I used the 7 Stages that were developed by Barry Reisberg, M.D., clinical Director of the New York University School of Medicine's Silberstein Aging and Dementia Research Center. We simply had to have some way to measure Carol's benchmark with the disease when we spoke to others, and this seemed to work well for us. We found it important when you talk to others to establish a benchmark of terms so that everyone can relate to what point your loved one is at. When we began the Alzheimer's topic with someone we would first point out that there are "7 stages".

During the day I had many opportunities to bring up the topic of Alzheimer's with people who I had conversations with. Chiefly this was during breaks, and lunch hours at my office. I learned a great deal from these conversations, as well as from the information that I read on the internet. When the home nurses came by at Carol's doctors request, we asked many questions and learned a lot about the disease in that manner. It was during one of the home nurses visits that the conversation came around to Carol's migraine headaches that she had in her youth. I asked her if anyone else in her family had migraine headaches, and she said that her brother Leonard did. Not long after this it dawned on me that Carol and Leonard had something else in common: they had both developed Alzheimer's Disease. With that thought in mind, I asked those at my office if by chance their relative had migraine headaches in their youth. Of the seven people who I talked with about AD, six said that there was a history of migraine headaches and one didn't know. Now, I want to reiterate that I'm not a Doctor; I'm just bringing this apparent common denominator to your attention. Perhaps, it was nothing more than a mere coincidence. Yet, I wouldn't rule out a link here... would you? It would be worth a mention for reference to your family physician if you think appropriate.

All things considered, I would strongly suggest that you begin your Memory Book no later than the middle of Stage 3. It is at this point where a decreased ability begins to remember some of your immediate family member's names. At least that's the way it was for Carol. However, we were lucky and learned of Carol's Alzheimer's before this time. Consequently, I was able to sit with Carol quite often and she was able to identify the people in the older family photographs, which were to be used later in her Memory Book. Carol had out lived her five brothers, and five sisters, so she was the last person who would be able to identify the people in the old photos. I learned this was really essential for those photographs, which I found in boxes around the house. Some of the photos were saved and passed down from generation to generation from the late 1800's!

When we became alerted to Carol's condition my wife and I had some decisions to make. Since Carol didn't want to leave her home where she lived for over 30 years, and move in with us, my wife and I decided to sell our home and build additional rooms on to Carol's house. This way we would be readily available to help her with her daily needs as her condition progressed. We didn't really know about Alzheimer's at the time, or how living with someone with Alzheimer's would directly affect our lives. When we decided to build the addition we just felt that it was "the right thing to do". Quite frankly, the observations which resulted in the development of the Memory Book would never have come to pass unless the experiences unfolded just the way they did. It brings to mind a prayer which someone once gave me that:

May today there be peace within you;
May you trust God that you are exactly where you are meant to be;
May you not forget the infinite possibilities that are born of faith;
May you use those gifts that you have received,
and pass on the love that has been given to you;
May you be content knowing you are a child of God.
Let this presence settle into your bones;

And allow your soul the freedom to sing, dance, praise and love;
It is there for each and every one of us.

Why was our decision the "right thing to do"? To answer this question we would both have to ask ourselves what led us to this inner belief. As for myself, I've had experience taking care of my elderly father and a terminally ill mother until they both passed on. I know that being a caregiver will make a person think about their own mortality, and I learned this in my early teens 40 years ago. It requires some soul searching for sure. In my youth I did just that, and my soul searching has continued through the years. I had to explore some ethical and spiritual concepts to try and understand the reality of death in my immediate family, particularly in my youth. Here I will share with you what I've learned as it applies to spirituality, and Alzheimer's Disease. Maybe it will help you cope with the reality of the situation, and the core of the matter.

All the major religions of the world recognize an essential element to humankind as being the soul. Again, it is said by these same religions that the human soul is already in a perfect condition. This seems to be supported pretty well in various scriptures. Over the course of time, I have also learned that there is one thing that we acquire while living that we *do take with us upon our death*, and that one thing is our personality. The personality that we develop, while living through all our various experiences, is actually an attribute of our own soul. In my opinion, the development of our personality is the reason that we are born into the world as a living soul. To have all the many lifelong experiences certainly shapes our personality, and in this way a person is always "becoming".

You are not the same person you were yesterday, last week, or last year. The task is to focus on recognizing the inner urges of our soul, and thereby evolve our personality. If we abide by these urges and govern our conduct by them, our personality goes through a transition and becomes, as they say, more "enlightened". So we actually do not evolve the soul, but we do evolve our personality which is striving to become attuned with the good nature of our inner most soul. It is with this idea that we find the prompting of the soul through a person's intuition. It was our intuition that said: "it's the right thing to do". Well, that's the shortened version of the wisdom that I've come to learn through the years. It makes sense to me at least.

With Alzheimer Disease the brain is affected. I've learned that the brain is the only organ of the body through which all the emotions, and desires, are consciously realized and find their power to function or be displayed outwardly. Alzheimer's Disease injures the functioning of the brain so that it affects the conscious, objective realization of facts or impressions, but that is all. Alzheimer's Disease may prevent the path which leads from the inner subconscious to the outer communication and motor skills, but such shutting off of this free passage of thought does not destroy the thought. Keep that in mind. Although the memory is stifled and made nonmanifest by this disease does not prove that memory resides in the flesh and bones of the human body. Paralysis may make mute and inactive every physical faculty and muscle of the human body to the extent where no sign or signal of intelligence may be expressed, but the mind will continue to think and have within its chambers many thoughts unable to manifest objectively. The personality is still within the body learning from each daily experience thelessons of the day. Again, this is just my opinion, but it makes sense to me.

Although neither my wife nor I are doctors we lived 7 days a week for about 5 years with Carol. You might call this our medical internship. Again, I can only advise on my observations and the conditions as they appeared to me during this time period. As Carol's condition progressed we tried hiring in-home nurse's, and having the immediate family come by to sit with Carol while my wife and I were at work. There seemed to be value in both of these approaches, as far as having a support network in place. Our concern was that Carol should not be left alone for two good reasons. First, she had good days and bad days. It's always better to have help, and insure Carol's safety so that she would remember to eat and take her medications. Second, in some states if you leave an Alzheimer's patient alone, no matter what stage they are in, and some tragic accident occurs you may be held libel... even if you don't live with the Alzheimer's patient. According to some of the conversations I've had with people whose loved ones have Alzheimer's, the courts can map together all kinds of issues if given encouragement. Some of the stories are a bit frightening to say the least. We felt we were doing the right thing, and followed our hearts.

It is from the personal experience of living together on a day by day basis, that I witnessed something which seemed to improve, at least in some small way, the quality of alertness and enthusiasm in Carol. It seemed to me that on the days I went over photographs with Carol that her mind seemed to focus better, and then maintain that focus for many hours thereafter. Yes, my review of the photographs with her actually seemed to stimulate her thinking process. She clearly appeared to remain alert afterward, which led to her actively engaging in domestic activity around the house. Sometime this resulted in odd things ending up in the refrigerator.

Witnessing firsthand the transitions which took place with this dreaded disease was really overwhelming for both my wife and me. I cringe to think that in the very near future there is a potential for a significant amount of people in the "baby boomer" generation to develop Alzheimer's. Yet, according to the World Health Organization dementias exceeded twelve million in 2008, and it has a projected 3.4% annual increase to about 14.3 million in 2013. Wikipedia's section on epidemiology states that "among people aged 65, two to three percent show signs of the disease, while up to fifty percent of people aged 86 have symptoms of Alzheimer's. Every five years after the age of 65, the probability of having the disease doubles". So let's hope someone finds a cure soon. Until that time, perhaps utilizing a tool such as a Memory Book will provide a stimulating activity that will enhance cognitive performance.

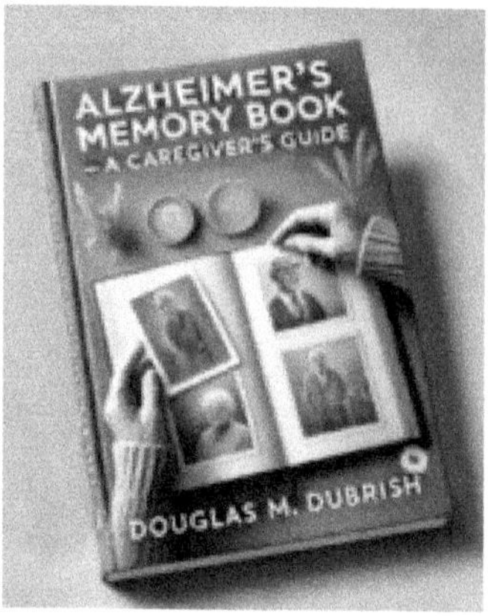
ALZHEIMER'S
MEMORY BOOK
– A CAREGIVER'S GUIDE
DOUGLAS M. DUBRISH

Chapter 2

Getting Started

Since the first permanent photograph was made in 1826, by French inventor Joseph Nicephore Niepce, photographs have stimulated the imagination. That stimulation is just what seems to be necessary for Alzheimer's patients to exercise their minds and utilize their memories.

Unlike the scrapbooking phenomenon of recent day, when you develop your "Alzheimer's Memory Book" I suggest that you really keep things simple in nature. The pages should be simple, and soothing to look at. They should not be loud with color, or busy with a lot of pattern like scrapbooks. Remember that your goal is to exercise the minds ability for remembering, and not to dazzle, or overpower someone's senses with color and pattern. Keeping it simple means: keeping it pleasant to the eye of the beholder. In this way I found that an elderly mind will remain focused on the photograph itself which is the goal.

The intent of the photograph is to stimulate memory, which in turn should provide conversation about the content of the photo, or perhaps provide new thought about some other topic. I noticed that as Carol progressed with Alzheimer's she frequently refrained from participating in conversations that were taking place around her. Maybe this was because if more than one conversation was going on she became very confused. So, you might want to keep that in mind as a caregiver when visiting. Remember, one conversation at a time.

Socialization skills seem to diminish as the mind begins a "withdraw" and Alzheimer's progresses. I mention this because it's natural if there are others around, when you are talking about the photographs, for them to engage in conversation more readily than the person with Alzheimer's. Insure everyone participates in the discussion about the pictures. A good "healthy conversation" goes a long way with Alzheimer's patients.

The purpose of your "Alzheimer's Memory Book" is to inhibit or delay the minds "withdraw" by using the photographs to stimulate memory and conversation. This will exercise the thinking process itself. Reminiscing in this way is important. In fact, the professionals actually gave this a name: "reminiscence therapy". According to Wikipedia the term "Reminiscence Therapy", called RT for short, is defined in that it "involves the discussion of past experiences individually or in a group, many times with the aid of photographs, household items, music and sound recording, or other familiar items from the past."

In your Alzheimer's Memory Book be sure to use only photographs that can provide a positive, uplifting memory as you sort and begin to design your book. You should want the individual to look back on life with a sense of gladness, and you should always want to leave a positive outcome while reminiscing. Try and provide a sense of fulfillment about life, as you decide upon the photos to use. This way the individual can accept their eventual death with a sense of dignity. Yes, death is something that we try not to think of. However, that's something you will have to come to terms with. Also, I recommend to avoid being confrontational, or arguing about any kind of facts related to the photographs. Instead, respond in an agreeable way. Remember that agitation, anxiety, anger, and depression are behavioral symptoms with AD, and you do not want to contribute to those symptoms.

With this in mind I would like to mention a few things about discussing the "news" when you're visiting. Try to remember when you're talking to someone with AD that "news" is an abbreviation. It stands for **N**egative **E**motional **W**orthless **S**tories as far as Alzheimer's patients are concerned. Actually, it should stand for that anytime. It is said that our brains have a "negativity bias" where we have a built in "greater sensitivity to unpleasant news". Research has apparently demonstrated that "our brain reacts more strongly to stimuli it deems negative. That is, there is a greater surge of electrical activity [in the cortex where the magnitude of information processing takes place]. Thus, our attitudes are more heavily influenced by downbeat news than good news." Many people start their normal day listening to the "magnitude" of news from their television or radio as they prepare to leave for work. Every day, every week, every month, and every year after year after year they listen to the morning "negative" news. What kind of peace of mind does that provide? The fact is the media are masters of disseat. They want to emotionally turn your mind towards disaster so they can sell those commercials to you while you're glued waiting on yet more negative news. And, if they get their facts wrong, which they do frequently, you will rarely if ever hear a correction. A case in point is the fact that: "There is no evidence that depression is caused by low serotonin". Rather than a chemical imbalance, resulting in depression may be caused by *prolonged stress...* from watching and listening to the NEWS! Please remember that *getting the story correct is not part of the news media's mission!* They know that you have a "weakness" towards negative news. They have been manipulating and exploiting you for years! I would strongly urge you not to bring up negative emotional worthless stories (NEWS) when you visit someone with AD. Remember that agitation, anxiety, anger, and depression are behavioral symptoms with AD, and you do not want to contribute to those symptoms by discussing negative news, or negative information regarding another family member's health. It's bad enough that in nursing homes across the country you will find the elderly in the "day rooms" with a television on with the local NEWS. I think they should be watching The Learning Channel, Animal Planet, Travel Channel, Discovery Channel, or something that ***would not*** give them a daily exposure to calamity on TV. Again, I'm not a Doctor. I just felt it was my duty to mention these things. I just recall a famous man who once said: "What is required of us now is a new era of responsibility – a recognition, on the part of every American, *that we have duties to ourselves*, our nation, and the world..." Certainly with this thought in mind we move forward, and try to reconcile those short comings we may witness. Perhaps, over time a more positive atmosphere will develop in the nursing home communities from those who visit them and see the shortcomings.

Keep in mind, that on the average, a person lives about 5 years after being diagnosed with Alzheimer's. A person may have had Alzheimer's for as long as 20 years, but only recently had it diagnosed since the symptoms began to show. That person with Alzheimer's just might be you someday. So be agreeable, and extend the kindnesses to them that you would have extended to you in the future.

Our experience as caregivers indicated that Carol's parents, and childhood experiences, seemed to last the longest in memory. This seems to conform well to one of the indicators provided in the Stage 5 characteristics. Consequently, when developing your Memory Book keep in mind that your format should be a sequence of pictorial events, starting from birth to present day. I found this to be a helpful and essential concept when recalling memories, and stories, related to the pictures. Rather than to jump around from childhood to adulthood then back to childhood, it seemed easier for Carol to transition from childhood memories gradually into her early adulthood, and then beyond. Otherwise there seemed to be a lot of confusion trying to recall the events in her memory. The goal here is to reinforce the individual's memory of their life's journey, from childhood into adulthood. In effect you are guiding that person sequentially along a journey through time which explores their lifelong memories in a chronological order. Health care professionals call the older memories in a person's life: episodic memory.

In late Stage 4 I found the Memory Book idea to really show its value. Carol was still living with us during this time. In viewing pictures over and over I found some memory improvement as each episode in Carol's life was recalled and briefly relived. If she didn't recall a picture we would move forward in the book, then go back to the photo and she was then apt to remember some detail. It was like the missing memory snapped into place. Again, you might find the improved retention to be short lived, but the uplifting effect which it has on the person with Alzheimer's will be worth it. Improving their quality of life is a "one day at a time" achievement.

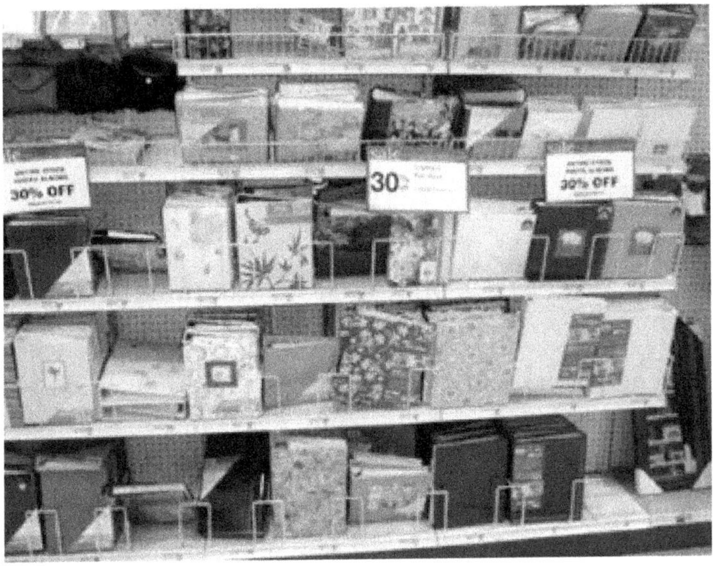

Common department store display of photograph books

To begin your Alzheimer's Memory Book please understand, that this doesn't have to be an expensive purchase. A photography book with 10 heavy paper inserts, with the capacity of 20 top loading pages, will provide plenty of room for your photographs. This type of photography book is available at most department stores, and would be durable enough, economical, and serve well for the situation. Often times you can find these items on sale.

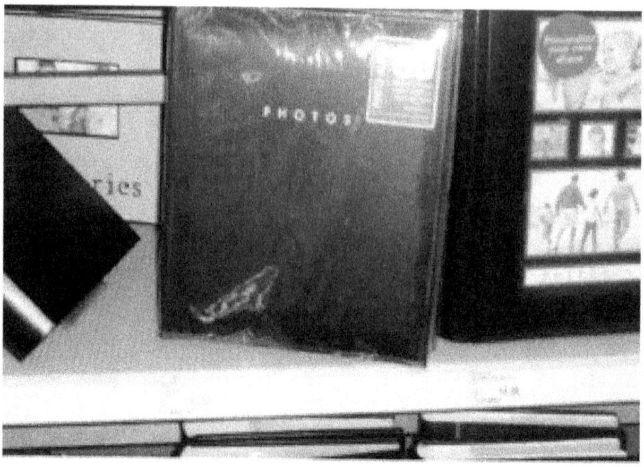

Inexpensive photograph book suitable
for your "Memory Book"

Keep in mind that the idea is not to swamp the individual with pictures, but to provide an opportunity for the memory to do its job of remembering. Having too many photographs to review may become taxing, tiring, and defeat the purpose. This may become more apparent during early Stage 6 when there is a disruption in the normal sleeping pattern. The elderly person may just fall asleep at mid day while you're talking to them. As a caregiver keep that in mind. You can always change the pictures in the book from time to time in order to challenge, and wake up the latent memory. That fresh challenge may promote improved mental health, in my opinion. Even if this event is a short term one.

Chapter 3

Segments of Time

Your "Alzheimer's Memory Book" should be segmented into time periods for easier memory recall. I considered the memory as being compartmentalized and developed the Memory Book into various periods of life accordingly. This certainly appeared to provide optimal results when the Memory Book was reviewed.

For a 20 page layout I would recommend three pages, of 3 photos each, which are to be divided into seven time periods of a person's life. By allowing for nine photographs for each of these time periods we increase the AD patients likelihood of recalling past events in a systematic methodical way. I found that if the photographs were arranged from top to bottom, in the manner indicated

below, the viewing pattern seemed to flow easily especially for an elderly eye to follow.

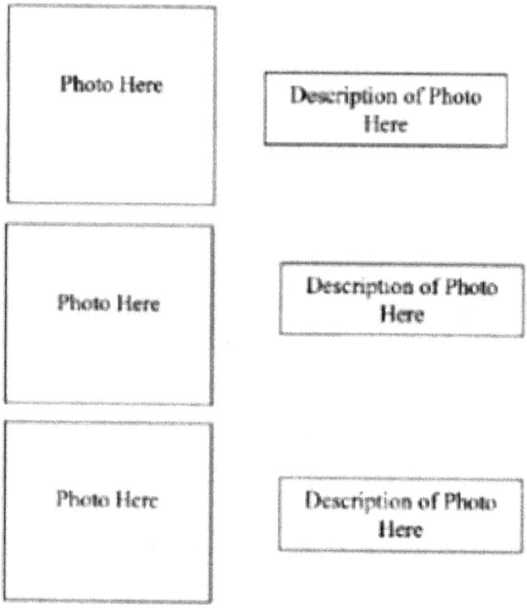

Page Diagram

Keep in mind that most families have elders who

remember rather clearly the events of the early nineteen hundreds, and who knew family members that reached back to the late eighteen hundreds. Passed on from their parents and grandparents many elders have acquired photographs, letters and family keepsakes that they have carefully stored in shoeboxes, envelopes and files. Perhaps this is the situation with the individual you are doing the Alzheimer's Memory Book for. It was certainly the situation for me.

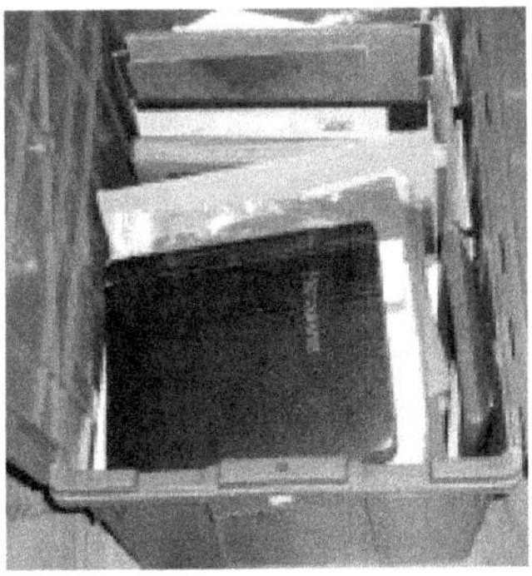

Photographs saved from the late 1800's to the late 1900's

These photographs may have been placed in closets, basements, and garages, with the very best of intentions, to be reviewed, sorted, and shared when that person found time to organize them at a later date. Yet, going into any antique shop anywhere in our country we find countless boxes of ancestral photographs, set out for sale, with nameless faces of forgotten people. This consequence is the result of good intentions that were never realized and fulfilled. You can make it happen!

The time is now if you want to identify any of those old pictures, which are lacking an identifying note on the reverse side. This might be "the last" opportunity to identify people, develop a pictorial biography, or even family history, since living memory of these people and events might soon be lost. By learning of details connected to the photos you might also inspire continued family traditions by connecting today's descendants directly with the lives of their forefathers. This is food for thought, and good food for the mind of a person with AD to review with you.

It isn't necessary to specify in the book the different time periods unless you feel compelled to. The ability to smoothly move through the book, and allow the memory to recall each photo, is the basic reason for compiling the photographs in a chronological order. Next to the photographs you should put a small message, or caption about the photo just as a reference to encourage the conversation regarding the particular event depicted in the picture. Yes, this will take a little time to complete. You have the time, they don't.

I found the following to be a good framework for developing the Memory Book system, and expanding the topics of conversation. There isn't a hard and fast rule except to try and find the earliest photograph and work towards the present day. Here's

the format I used and would highly recommend:

Section 1) from Birth to 3 years – Infancy to Toddler

Section 2) from 3 to 7 years – Play Years

Section 3) from 7 to 11 years – Elementary School Age

Section 4) from 11- 18 years – Adolescence

Section 5) from 19 to 40 – Young Adulthood

Section 6) from 40 to 65 – Middle Adulthood

Section 7) from 65 and beyond – Late Adulthood

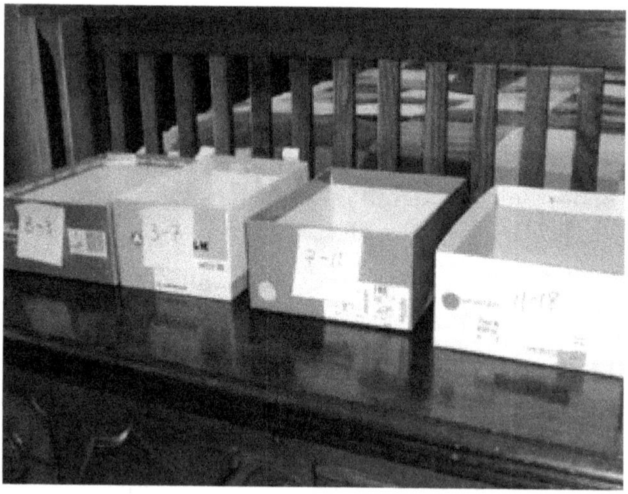

Labeled boxes help sort photographs
according to a person's age

Section 1)- from birth to 3 years. Very few people can remember prior to the age of 3, especially in late adulthood. However, if photos exist they should likely be included, since they might bring up discussion on some other topic. Again, this would allow the memory to be exercised. You will likely be going back at least 65 years in the chronology of the photographs selected for your book. Because, after all, the early onset of Alzheimer's disease could begin when a person reaches their mid 60s.

Sometimes photo's are taken when a special event is achieved that might be memorable. For example: if a child of 3 swims in an ocean it would be inevitable that they would receive a gulp of salt water in the mouth. That nasty taste of salt might be an event that they would remember throughout their lives, since they had only known fresh water. Then after the swim the child might wonder why they would have to "shower off" since they were just in the water. Both of these experiences being new, and unusual, an elderly person might be inclined to still remember many decades later. Perhaps, in their early years they attended an amusement park, or a county fair that they would remember. Any first time occasions of this nature might be memorable ones. Certainly, you can be flexible. Just include additional photographs for the next section if photos for this time period are lacking.

Section 2) -from 3 to 7 years. In this age bracket a person's first time memories would be on the increase. A school picture would bring discussion on the name of the person's first teacher. Surprisingly many people remember the name of their very first school teacher. Also, if there is seasonal change in the area where a person grew up then a discussion on winter activities like ice skating, or sledding might be topics for discussion that would jog the childhood memories.

Section 3)-from 7 to 11 years. During this period young people are generally eager to learn and accomplish more complex skills like reading, writing, and telling time. Maybe during this time segment there were awards that the individual won in their early school years that would be memorable. One of the things that were very popular many years ago was a "spelling bee". Sometimes the awards came in the form of dictionaries with the person's name engraved on the cover. This would certainly be a memorable event. Other memorable events could be a baptism, or confirmation at a church, or someone's wedding they went to. Again, outdoor sports activities may have increased to include a wider range with seasonal activity like swimming, baseball, or fishing.

Section 4) -from 11- 18 years – During this segment of a person's life their appearance to others becomes very important. While in school many people would join a sport team, the band, or another activity which would increase their socialization with others. In the latter part of High School people began to think about an occupational identity. If the individual was born in a foreign country it could be this period of time they may think about future immigration, or even naturalization associated with an upper lever education in a foreign country.

Section 5)-from 19 to 40 – During this period of young adulthood an individual normally wants to blend in with friends, and develop commitments with others. A person's higher education, occupation, and financial interests become increasingly important during this period. Also, an individual may join the Armed Services, professional societies, become a member of a variety of team sports, and begin to travel, or enjoy increasing recreational activities like water skiing, diving, canoeing, boating or golf. Marriage and raising a family also begins during this period, and is the inspiration for a multitude of pictures and family experiences.

Section 6)- from 40 to 65 – Middle Adulthood – Concern for a person's extended family appears to grow as the reality of aging begins to set in during this period. Grandchildren arrive and become an important part of life. Pictures are taken at many holidays and birthday celebrations which could be used in the Memory Book.

Section 7) -from 65 and beyond – Late Adulthood – This is a time when a person will look back on life and the many paths they traveled. A new sense of integrity and readiness for whatever may lay ahead normally develops during this period. A sense of fulfillment about life, and the overall experiences that were lived.

You can place the photographs on the adhesive page, or use the special tapes or settings available, and then print a caption to place directly to the right of the photo. There are other options. One option is to scan the photographs into your computer data base, and then enter the photo in a text box on to a blank "word" document. By creating another text box, immediately to the right of your picture, you can provide for the caption with this method. It would be easy to expand, or change the photographs from time to time. You can save each page, and then print it to construct the Memory Book. Yes, you can certainly expand on this idea as well. By scanning the photographs you would be preserving the photo image from deterioration in a box, or the yellowing process as the photo ages. Below is an example of this type of scanned database process.

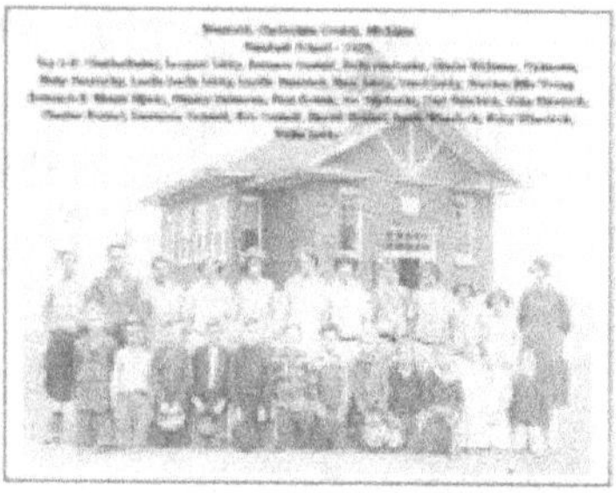

The school house
1925

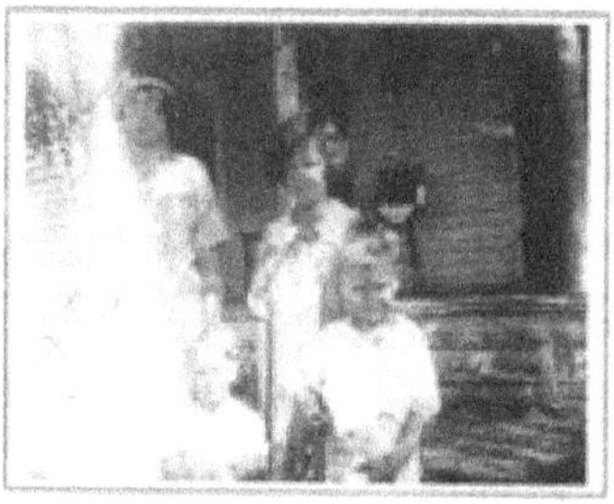

On the farm porch
1928

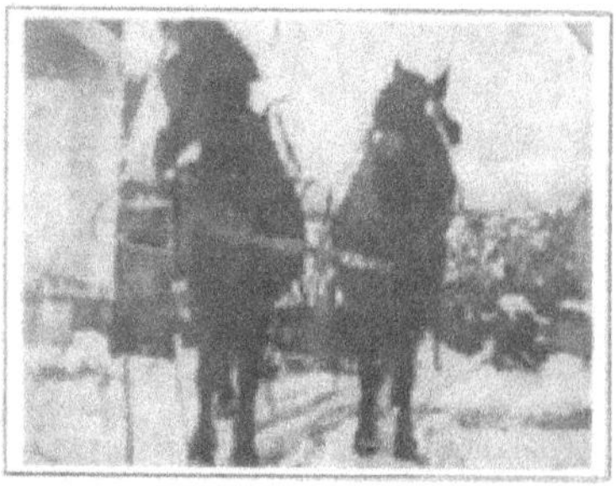

The family horse team
Prince & Doll
1928

An example of a page format with captions

Chapter 4
Conversation

The person before you, who has Alzheimer's Disease, is going through some very significant changes, and they might not be able to realize these changes themselves. At times, it will be hard for you to come to grips with the reality of this situation. Although in the past they may have been able to identify people in photographs instantly, you will find that this ability will slowly fade. There will come a time when even your own identity will be unknown to them. Although, they will likely know that yours is a familiar face. Watching someone progress with Alzheimer's Disease involves a lot of understanding, and compassion, on the part of the caregiver. And, as a caregiver you will likely become psychologically drained and perhaps depressed as you witness this disease progress. I'm not going to dwell on this, because in all likelihood if you're reading this book you are aware of these aspects already. But, if you haven't read up on Alzheimer's Disease on the various internet websites, or checked out a book about the disease from your local library, you need to do so now.

If you're a child, or close grandchild of the person with Alzheimer's then you will be overwhelmed. Your emotional attachment will be very hard to deal with, and at times you may have difficulty thinking of things to talk about. The fact is: the stress of the whole situation can really leave you speechless. Keep in mind that the individual with Alzheimer's may seem subdued and withdrawn. That's part of the disease. Your challenge is to cheer that person up with a positive attitude, which can improve their quality of life for that day or at least during the time you spend with them. That's another reason the Alzheimer's Memory Book is so important. The Memory Book provides a focal point of activity when the situation may otherwise seem to be overwhelming to you.

With that in mind try to remember the basics: who, what, where, why, and when, as you look through the pictures together. Although "you" may already know the: who, what, where, why, and when of the pictures, and perhaps you just went through the pictures two days ago, keep in mind that you are in effect an "exercise instructor". As you point to a person in a picture you are exercising your companion's memory. This is similar to a much slower version of "Flash Cards" that you may have played in your own youth. Also, keep in mind as you exercise their memory, this may help slow the cognitive decline that comes with Alzheimer's. Here are some helpful tips...

"Who" questions can make a person think of another individual or their family relationship to the individual in the picture. When you point to a person ask the question: "Who is that again?", even though you may already know the answer. Your goal is to try to create a dialog and encourage their memory to remember.

"What" questions will seek to understand what really happened, or give you the meaning of something. As you point to the person in the picture ask: "What did he do for a living?" Also, be prepared to redirect the person's attention should a photograph bring back a negative memory. Quickly move on to the next picture, and remove the unwanted picture as soon as possible.

"Where" type of questions will help to establish a location, or place of an event that is seen in the photograph. Such as: "Where did they get married at? Or, where did that family reunion take place?"

"Why" type of questions will help determine the motivation which influenced something. Maybe a question like: "Why did aunt Carols pie crusts always look, and taste better than everyone else's?"

"When" questions will help to place the photo in its proper time period. Maybe if the year can't be determined you might be able to ask about the season of the year that the photo was taken. This might help in identifying the year and bring a recollection back to mind. Below is the book which I developed.

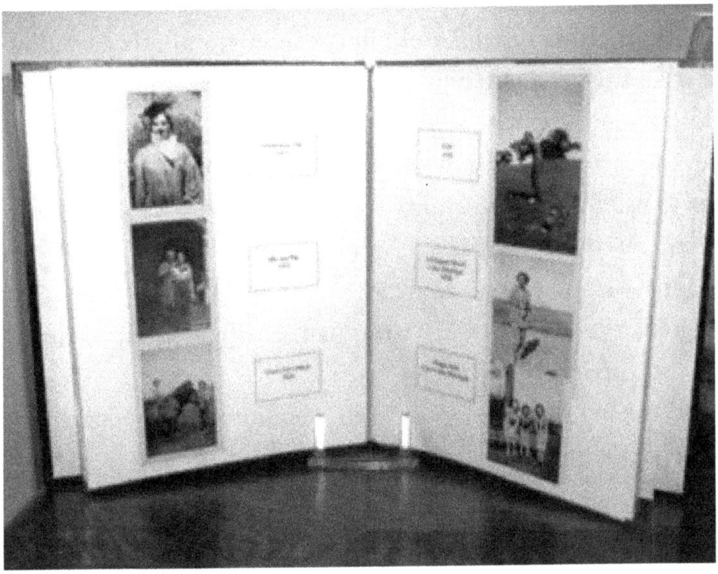

The main thing is to stimulate conversation, and to exercise the memory. That's your goal!

Checklist

Locate a work area which can be used temporarily for your Memory Book project. It can be an unused guest bedroom or a floor area of a less utilized room.

Locate photographs to be used in Memory Book.

Gather photographs into designated work area.

Acquire photographs from relatives if available.

Photographs should be copied before returning to owner if appropriate.

Sort photographs.

Shoeboxes identified with the various time periods.

Pile the photographs with a label nearby indicating time periods.

Photograph Selection

Identify the photographs that you feel might be best to create a conversation. Think of what questions you might ask that would be the happiest for the person to recall.

Utilize your Memory Book

Review the effects of how the conversation went.

Try to use the same Memory Book content on your next visit.

Compare the two visits to see if recollection had improved

Modify Memory Book content

Change the photographs to enhance different memories of the various time periods.

Scan the pages to keep in your computer for compiling into a pictorial family history is desired

Chapter 5

Heritage Inquiry

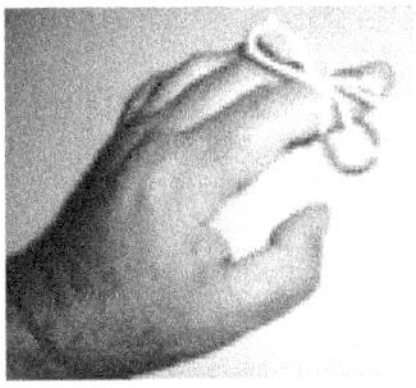

Since people afflicted with Alzheimer's disease are elderly there is also a great loss of family heritage that coincides with the condition. To help preserve family traditions and strengthen family ties try to document oral tradition for future generations before it becomes lost. Sometimes the simplest questions can be a real source of family lore that will inspire and intrigue others. Preserving memories can be a positive bonding experience between the Alzheimer's sufferers, future generations, and the caregiver. Perhaps, you might acquire enough information to create a book and dedicate it to your loved one or friend.

To help you along the conversational avenue are the following questions that might spark fresh insight, kinship ties, family lore, and the preservation of your heritage. Remember, when your friend with Alzheimer's begins to get tired you should stop and save your other questions for another day.

When and where were you born?

Where did you go to Elementary School? High School?

Did you have an after school or summer job during your youth?

What did you like about it?

What did you dislike about it?

What were you paid for your work?

How did you spend the money you made?

Did you have any hobbies growing up?

Did you join any youth groups like scouts, 4-H Clubs, or engage in sports?

What kind of new invention impressed you when you were growing up?

Did you do anything special for your childhood birthdays?

Growing up did you have any routine chores around your home that were your responsibility?

What memorable things did you do with your father or mother?

What were the names of your four grandparents?

Do you know where they were born?

Have you heard the legend of where the family originally came from?

What was the house like that you grew up in?

During the religious holidays how did you decorate your childhood home?

What kind of family tradition do you recall was unique during the holidays for your family?

Did you continue this tradition into your home as an adult?

What other major holidays did you celebrate in your home during your childhood?

What was your favorite food during the holidays, and how was it prepared?

What was the most memorable thing that happened during your teenage years?

Did you go to College? Trade School? Graduate School? Military?

What was the name of the College that you attended? What was your major?

Which military service were you in?

Where were you stationed?

As a young adult what occupation were you in?

Did you choose the occupation or happen into it?

What did you especially like about the job?

What did you dislike about the job?

How much did you earn when you started?

Where did you live when you were a young adult?

What kind of car did you first buy?

When you had an opportunity did you do any traveling during your youth?

Did you start any new hobbies when you were a young adult?

What kind of historical events did you witness during your young adult years?

Did you have the occasion to meet anyone that you would consider famous?

How did you and your spouse meet?

What do you feel attracted you to each other?

Where did you your wedding take place?

What are the names of your children?

How did you pick the children's names?

What was one of the funniest things that each child did growing up?

What religion did you become a member of?

What do you like about it?

Did you participate in any church social activities?

Did your children become members of the same church?

As an adult, what one invention do you recall being invented -during your life- that people take for granted in the present day?

Chapter 6

Further Reading

National Institute of Mental Health. Depression. Retrieved June 14, 2008, from Http://nimh.nih.gov/health/topics/depression/index.shtml

National Institute on Aging. Alzheimer's. Retrieved June 14, 2008, from http://www.nia.nih.gov/alzheimers/publications/unraveling/part3/causes.htm.

Silberstein Aging and Dementia Research Center. Alzheimer's. Retrieved June 14, 2008, from http://aging.med.nyu.edu/

Staff, P.T. (1992). Armchair Shell Shock. Psychology Today, Article ID 1880, retrieved December 31, 2008, from http://www.psychologytoday.com/articles/pto-19920501-000008.html

Marano, Hara Estroff (2003). Why We Love Bad News. Psychology Today. Article ID 2802, retrieved December 31, 2008, from http://www.psychologytoday.com/articles/pto-20030527-000004.html

Marano, Hara Estroff (1999). The Bad News Bias. Psychology Today Article 468, retrieved December 31, 2008, from http://psychologytoday.com/articles/pto-199990501-000012.html

Leo, J. and Lacasse, J.R. (2007) The Media and The Chemical Imbalance Theory of Depression. Retrieved December 31, 2008 from

http://psychrights.org/articles/
leolacassemadiaandchemicalimbalance.pdf

Dear Reader,

Thank you for choosing to read my book. I highly value your opinion! Please consider leaving a review. Your feedback helps others decide on their purchase. Your review makes a meaningful impact.

Thank you for your time and support!

Best regards,

Doug

Other books by Douglas M. Dubrish

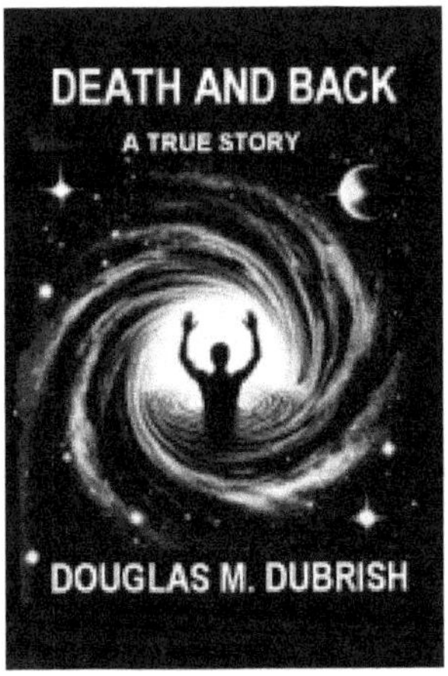

You might like this book because you've just lost someone close to you or you know someone who is terminally ill and you're looking for answers, comfort and reassurance. The author's unique journey is a testament to the power of near-death experiences, offering a rare glimpse into the realms beyond our understanding. As readers embark on this extraordinary voyage, they will witness a captivating blend of personal revelation, scientific exploration, and spiritual awakening.

Discover the secrets that individuals often choose to keep hidden, especially those who have encountered death. "Death and Back" sheds light on the reasons behind the silence surrounding near-death experiences, addressing fears of ridicule and societal judgment. The narrative also delves into the transformative impact such experiences can have on one's personality, demystifying the stigma associated with unconventional behavior.

Published: April 2020

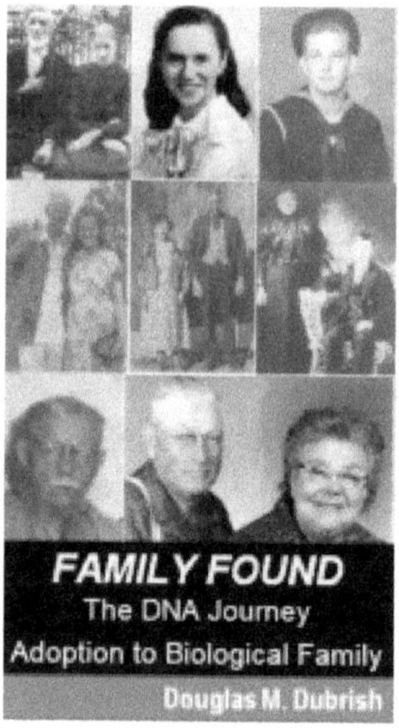

The book delves into the complexities of unraveling family secrets, questioning the authenticity of official documents, and the unexpected twists revealed through DNA testing. Explore his childhood discovery of adoption and the realization that the word "adopted" carried a weight he hadn't perceived as a young boy. The journey extends into adulthood, where genealogy and the pursuit of truth unfold, sometimes challenging the veracity of cherished family narratives.

Uncover the pitfalls and triumphs of the DNA testing journey, where conflicting information may surface, and unexpected relatives come to light. The story culminates in the discovery of long-lost siblings, the challenges of approaching family members as an "outsider," and the revelation that "trusted" state documents were not as accurate as believed.

Published: February 2022

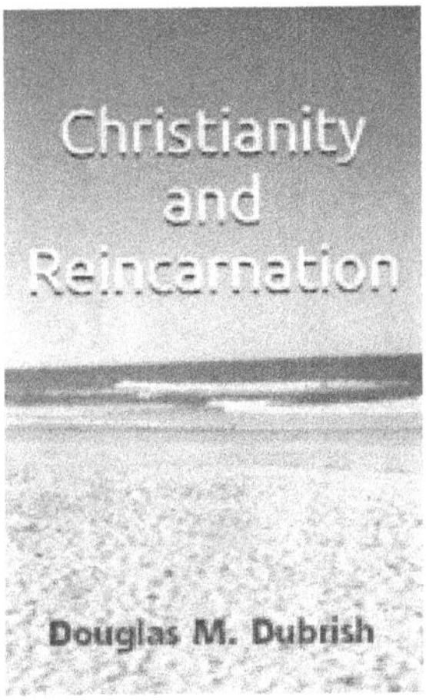

Dive into a captivating exploration of forgotten history with "Christianity and Reincarnation," a groundbreaking book that challenges conventional beliefs about Christianity and reincarnation. Discover the suppressed Doctrine of Reincarnation, once a core principle of the Catholic Church for 400 years, believed to have been taught by Jesus to his Apostles. Unravel the political intrigues that led to its removal in 543 A.D. and the subsequent omissions from the Bible by dedicated Catholic monks.

This eye-opening narrative delves into recent archaeological revelations, exposing the teachings of the Essene Community, the ancient sect to which Jesus and his family belonged. Unveil the hidden references to reincarnation deliberately excluded from the Bible by meticulous hand-copying over centuries. The book serves as a valuable resource for those seeking a comprehensive understanding of the Doctrine of Reincarnation and its significant role in the early years of Christianity.

Published: December 2022

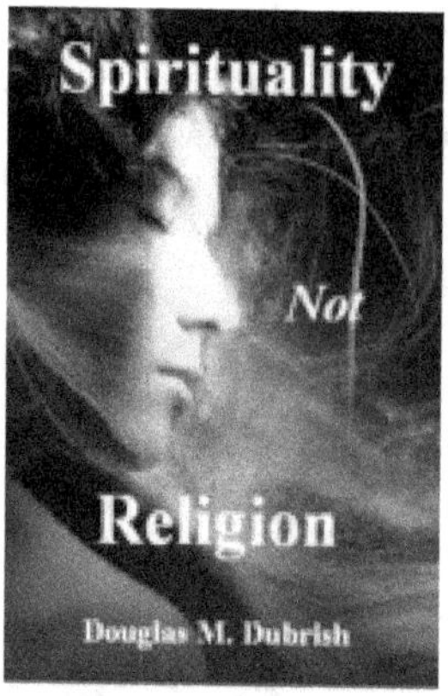

Embark on a captivating journey as the narrative unfurls a Cloth of Light, exploring the profound connections between the Shroud of Turin, the Sudarium of Oviedo, and residual atomic radiation images. In the pursuit of knowledge, the book skillfully draws upon the authoritative references of biblical texts, with the deciphering of the Rosetta Stone, which unlocks our own intellectual landscape.

In a poignant exploration, "Spirituality not Religion" weaves a tapestry of resilience in the face of adversity, uncovering the spirituality that perseveres even in the crucible of war. Through meticulous research, this book invites readers to ponder the profound mysteries that connect humanity's past, present, and eternal spirit in the new age.

Published: December 2023

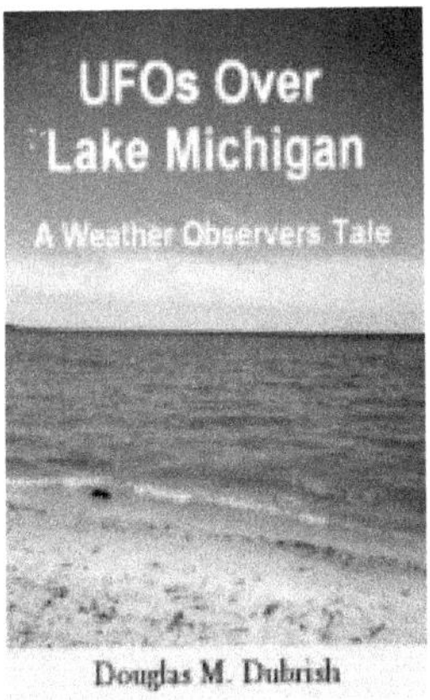

It has been just over 30 years since that unforgettable Tuesday night when multiple sightings of Unidentified Flying Objects were reported over the skies of Lake Michigan, just south of Muskegon. During the week beginning March 8th, 1994, over 300 accounts of UFO sightings were documented across Muskegon, Ottawa, Berrien, and Allegan counties in Lower Michigan.

UFO sightings over Lake Michigan were not uncommon at the National Weather Service Office in Muskegon. Every observer at the station witnessed these enigmatic lights, particularly during evening and midnight shifts. My own introduction to UFOs occurred not in Muskegon, but during my military service as an Air Traffic Controller in the U.S. Air Force. Stationed at Murphy Dome Air Force Site in Alaska in 1973, I observed unidentified flying objects over what is now known as the Alaskan Triangle.

Published: August 2024

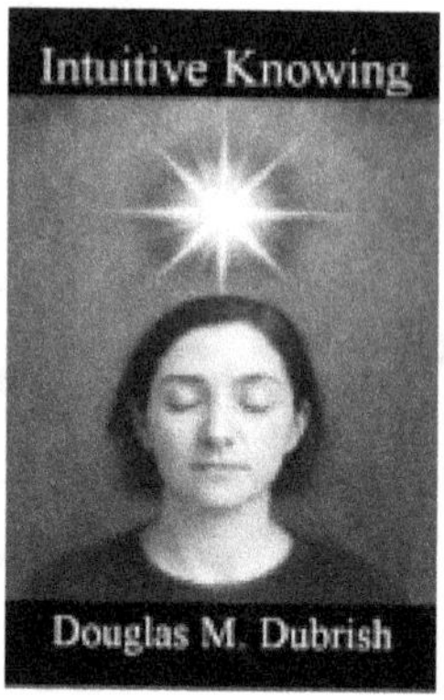

Intuition is not imagination, guesswork, or wishful thinking. It is the quiet, powerful voice within—a sacred sense of knowing that transcends logic and leads us toward truth, healing, and clarity.

Intuitive Knowing takes readers on a journey through ancient wisdom, personal insight, and modern reflections to rediscover the intuitive voice that lives inside us all. From the Eye of Horus in ancient Egypt to the teachings of Plato and Socrates, this book traces how intuition has been honored and forgotten—and how it now calls to be remembered.

Whether you've ignored your intuition for years or have always been quietly guided by it, this book invites you to reclaim the power of your sixth sense. Through practical insights and timeless teachings, *Intuitive Knowing* helps you understand that intuition is not a gift for a few—it's a universal faculty waiting to be awakened in all of us.

Published: August 2025

Family histories available

Ames Family History and Genealogy (2009)
Bays Family History and Genealogy (2021)
Bohy Family History and Genealogy (2005)
Cobb Family History and Genealogy
– English Roots Kentucky Branches (2024)
Dubrish Family Ancestry (1984)
Greuber Family History and Genealogy (2009)
Holmes Family in America (2006)
Jenkinson Family History and Genealogy (2000)
Liddy Family History and Genealogy (2006)
Mahaffey Family History and Genealogy (2009)
Sands Family History and Genealogy (2009)
Scheele family History and Genealogy (2012)
Smith Family History and Genealogy
- Kentucky Pioneers (2020)
Striebich Family History and Genealogy (2004)
Taylor Family History and Genealogy (2024)
Wedge Family History and Genealogy (2010)
Whitehead Family Heritage 1739 - 1939 (2002)
Woodworth Family History and Genealogy (2009)

Other books of interest

Christianity and Reincarnation (2021)

Death and Back - A True Story (2020)

Family Found – The DNA Journey (2022)

Spirituality Not Religion (2023)

Florida Keys Weather History (1987),

Hurricanes of the Lower and Middle Florida Keys (1985),

Our House Ghost - Selected Paranormal Incidents (2020),

Pioneer America - Recipes and Herbs from the 1800s (1988),

The Alzheimer's Memory Book - A Caregivers Guide (2008),

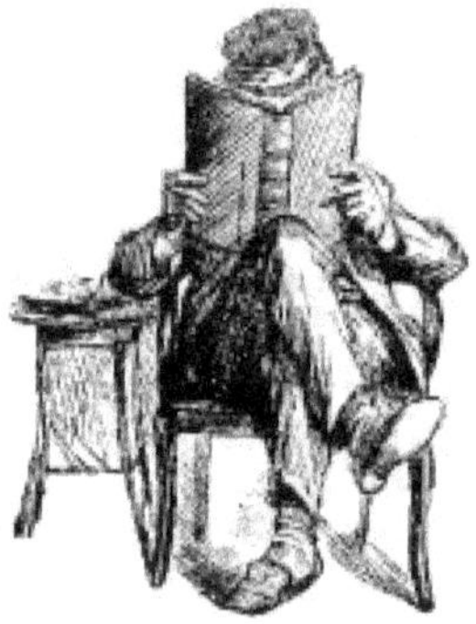

Don't miss out!

Visit the website below and you can sign up to receive emails whenever Douglas M. Dubrish publishes a new book. There's no charge and no obligation.

https://books2read.com/r/B-A-DFFAE-OKHNG

www.ingramcontent.com/pod-product-compliance
Lightning Source LLC
LaVergne TN
LVHW050344210926
848481LV00017B/1407